MIND YOUR IMMUNE SYSTEM

Your 21-Day Immune System Tracker Challenge

GLADYS GLOBAL

TABLE OF CONTENTS

INTRODUCTION

❝Health is wealth" is one of the common sayings that I grew up with, and that still retains its relevance around me to date. However, it is ironic to see how most of us pay keen attention to the building of wealth every day than helping our health. In the cause of chasing wealth, trying to keep our jobs or doing any other things that keep us relevant, we almost put our health in the balance every day. And while we do this, our health needs to get the treat that ensures our safety when our body is confronted by the enemy that has a goal to wreck our body.

Our bodies as carefully and wonderfully as they were created, they know when to react to what is happening in their environments as soon as possible, in such a way that the information we receive makes us call for medical assistance. The truth is that we don't know when the enemy of our body attacks, but we know when it comes in but how we have prepared our bodies' security determines what happens, and that is why we have this title to deal with today. The securities are known as the Immune system.

IMMUNE SYSTEM

The immune system is a very complex and well-coordinated network of specialized tissues, cells, and organs in the body, working as the defense of the body against several infections that may attack the body. One amazing thing about the immune system is that it keeps the historical record of every microbe, which is also known as germ, that has been previously defeated so that such germs maybe swiftly recognized in case it attacks the body again then the system can ensure its speedy destruction. When a germ invades successfully, that is when we become sick.

There are three types of immunity in Humans which are: innate, adaptive, and passive:

Innate Immunity: This is a form of natural immunity that everyone is born with, and it ensures a type of general protection.

Our skins serve as a protector of our body from germs. When some certain aliens invade our body the immune system recognizes it.

Adaptive Immunity: It is a form of immunity that develops throughout our lives. It is either called Adaptive or Active Immunity, but we develop this form of immunity when we are either exposed to diseases or when we get immunization against them using vaccines.

Passive Immunity: It is a type of immunity that we can say to have been "borrowed" from a different source to last for a short period of time. Antibodies in a mother's breast milk provide her baby with short time immunity to diseases that the mother has been exposed to is an example of Passive Immunity.

Weak Immune System

Someone's immune system may be declared as weak when the rate at which the person gets infection is frequently more than most other persons. We may also say an immune system is weak when it does not function the way it should work. This is not always a good situation because the treatment of those illnesses might be very difficult to come by. Some of the signs of a Weak Immune System can be a digestive issue, which may include loss of appetite, diarrhea, abdominal cramping, growth delay in infants and children, etc. You might have seen people with some of these signs;

however, the list below shows how the system might get to what it is in those whose immune system are not working well:

1. Primary Immune Deficiency: This is when the person is born with a weak Immune system.

2. Acquired Immune System: This happens when a disease has weakened a person's immune system.

3. Auto-immune Disease: In a situation like this, a person has an immune system that turns against him or her.

4. Over-active Immune System: In this situation, a person has an immune system that is too active.

VIRUSES

Viruses are tiny parasites that can be seen only with an electron microscope because they are much smaller than bacteria. They cannot grow well and reproduce outside any targeted body, which is generally referred to as the "host body." Viruses have built a reputation for being the cause of the disease's transmission from one person or organism to another.

In other words, viruses are contagious and often result in the death of the host body. The virus has a significant role, which is to deliver its DNA genome into the host cell so that the genome can be transcribed and translated by the host cell. The first thing viruses need is to access the inside of a host's body, which can happen through respiratory passages and open wounds. Insects can sometimes provide the mode of entry, but some viruses will hitch a ride in an insect's saliva and enter the host's body after the insect bites.

When a virus infects a person (host), it invades the cells of its host in order to survive and multiply. The moment it gets inside, the cells of the immune system cannot detect the virus and therefore do not know that the host cell is infected. To overcome this, cells will employ a system that allows them to show other cells what has invaded them. They, in turn, use molecules known as class I major histocompatibility complex proteins to display pieces of protein from inside the cell upon the surprise of the cell. If it is discovered that the cell is infected with a virus, these pieces of peptide will include fragments of proteins that the virus has made.

BACTERIA

Bacteria are single-celled microscopic organisms that grow excellently in different types of environments. This implies that they are organisms that can live in the soil, ocean, and inside the human gut. The relationship between humans and bacteria is very complex. Bacteria, sometimes, lend us a helping hand, in one way or the other, either by curdling milk into yogurt or helping with our digestion. In other cases, bacteria are so destructive, instigating diseases like pneumonia.

Moreover, bacteria are classified as organisms that have a simple internal structure that lacks a nucleus. It has been discovered through research that molecules on the surface of the spores are bound to molecules that are on the surface of the B cells. This binding then triggers the B cells to divide and multiply. These B cells are one of the major components of the immune system, and they produce the antibodies that fight harmful bacteria and viruses.

Building A strong Immune System

While it is a great idea to boost one's immunity totally, it is worth noting that the ability to do so may be difficult for several reasons. This is so because the immune system is a system, not a single entity that functions in isolation. It requires balance and harmony to perform well and there are still many things that researchers are yet to know all about the complexity and interconnectedness of the immune response. There are no direct, scientifically proven links between enhanced immune system function and lifestyle.

However, researchers are taking so much advantage of diet, age, psychological stress, exercise, and other immune response factors both in animals and humans. The effects of lifestyle on the immune system are fascinating and should be studied. As far as it stands, healthy-living strategies are generally an excellent way to start boosting one's immune system.

Something intriguing about life is that you will have to choose the way you would like to live it, which means you can choose to have a healthy life or an unhealthy one. Your first step in building a great immune system is by choosing a healthy way of life. There are proper health guidelines that can be taken towards keeping your immune system healthy and strong naturally if you can follow them. Healthy living strategies protect your body from different forms of assault from the environment and also make all parts of the body, and the immune system function better.

Below are the recommended guidelines for a good healthy lifestyle:

- Eat a diet high in fruits and vegetables.

- Do not smoke.

- Exercise regularly.

- Maintain a healthy weight.

- Avoid Alcohol.

- Get adequate sleep.

- Wash your hands frequently, and cooking meats thoroughly are some ways to avoid infection.

- Try to minimize stress.

The above list consists of things that are directly or indirectly supported in the Bible. So, if we eat the way God wants us to eat, we would build a strong immune system, and we would not be falling sick now and then. God has given us the body, and how we maintain it is in our hands. We can only live a life of purpose when we are in good health. Dear friend, you need to understand that God is interested in your well-being always. I Cor. 6:19-20 states: 19. Do you not know that your bodies are temples of the Holy Spirit, who is in you, whom you have received from God? You are not your own; 20. You were bought at a price. Therefore honor God with your bodies (NIV).

This portion of the Bible tells us how living a healthy life is one of the several ways to worship God, which is contrary to our daily opinion that we own our lives and bodies. This perspective of self-ownership has led countless to use their body simply the way they want. God has some amazing plans for our spirit, soul, and body, which are clearly expressed in Psalms 91:16, which states that "with long life I will satisfy him and show him my salvation."

Undoubtedly, it means that God did not put His precious breath in your body that it will not last long as He has desired. Remember that Jeremiah 29:11 says, "For I know the thoughts that I think toward you, saith the LORD, thoughts of peace, and not of evil, to give you an expected end" (KJV). This passage also has "God's know," but we need to note that this is God's agenda for every one created by Him. There is an end that God is expecting about your spirit, soul, and body, and we have a significant role to play before God can achieve that.

WHAT WE EAT

When God created man, the Bible says, He put him in a garden called Eden (Genesis 2:15); this suggests God's desire for good meals, especially vegetables and fruits. This type of meal has been consistently confirmed by researchers as a major ingredient for building a strong immune system. It has been proven beyond doubts that one kind of fruit or vegetable does not contain every nutrient needed to solidify the defense of our immune system. So, varieties are well recommended. Therefore, how often we consume them and the quality of what we consume matters a lot. In other words, your life has a considerable attachment to whatever you eat.

Having a deep understanding of what we consume and why we eat what we eat is crucial. At this point, I will give you a little breakdown of some foods. Any diet that you take, which is rich in vegetables and fruits, has the power to lower blood pressure. This type of diet also prevents some types of cancer and reduces the risk of having heart disease and stroke. The eyes and the digestive system also benefit as the diet ensures that they have less risk being attacked with illnesses particular to them. Its positive effect on blood sugar helps keep the appetite in check. When you consume non-starchy vegetables and fruits like pears, apples and green leafy vegetables help with shedding weight. The low glycemic loads in them can increase hunger when it prevents blood sugar spikes.

There are potentially hundreds of different plant compounds that are of great benefit to health that each of them has at least nine different families of fruits and vegetables that exist. To give your body the needed mix nutrients, please, try as much as you can to eat a variety of types and colors of produce to ensure a greater diversity of beneficial plant chemicals. At the same time, it also creates some fantastic meals that are appealing to the eye.

Focusing on building a healthy physical body and immune system by having a proper diet lets us balance it with spiritual food. Matthew 4:4 gives us an account of what Jesus said: ...it is written: Man shall not live by bread alone, but on every word that comes from the mouth of God (NIV). Daily feeding from God's word solidifies our relationship with God, boosts our faith to trust in His promises, and ultimately enhances our immune system significantly. We become what we read daily in the Bible, which has each of its words by God's inspiration. Let us consider what God said in Joshua 1:8 that we should "Keep this Book of the Law always on your lips; meditate on it day and night, so that you may be careful to do everything written in it. Then you will be prosperous and successful."

The prosperity that our souls enjoy can be balanced when our health is positively affected by it. John the Apostle has a beautiful admonition for us in 3 John 1:2 and the Amplified version of the Bible has it as "Beloved, I pray that in every way you may succeed and prosper and be in good health [physically], just as [I know] your soul prospers [spiritually]." Therefore, it is absolutely and dangerously insecure to pay more attention to either the spiritual or the physical. So, it is best when the two are well considered to be balanced.

When we get a balanced meal from the word of God daily, then we grow daily. Failure to eat daily from the Lord's dining table is total starvation for that period. God's word feeding per day is simply a balanced nutrient that keeps us safe from both physical and spiritual bacteria and viruses. From the spiritual, we control our physical health according to the word of God that we declare over ourselves and households. However, this should not be a yardstick for us to avoid good physical diets; both physical and spiritual meals must be balanced. 1 Timothy 4:8 teaches us that physical exercise is of some value for this life but spiritual exercise has all value for this life and eternal life.

While the natural diet ensures that our body is fit and well enough that our immune system can withstand infection and overcome them now, the system, however, becomes weaker as we grow older. Therefore, if we can put our mind in the spiritual diets, it covers us in this life and prepares our spirit man for the eternal life beyond the blue. Daily consumption of God's word strengthens our relationship with God and hides us from any form of attack more and more. When our spirit man has been continually fed, it daily becomes more like God. It will definitely shun some lifestyle that will make the physical and spiritual body vulnerable to attack.

Furthermore, Apostle Paul put it in a convincing manner in his letter to the Galatians in chapter 5:16-21 that "...walk by the Spirit, and you will not gratify the desires of the flesh. For the flesh desires what is contrary to the Spirit, and the Spirit, what is contrary to the flesh. They are in conflict with each other so that you cannot do whatever you want. But if you are led by the Spirit, you are not under the law. The acts of the flesh are obvious: sexual immorality, impurity and debauchery; idolatry and witchcraft; hatred, discord, jealousy, fits of rage, selfish ambition, dissensions, factions and envy; drunkenness, orgies, and the like. I warn you, as I did before, that those who live like this will not inherit the kingdom of God."

Overcoming Stress

One of the vital powers that God has given man is the power to decide or make a choice such that in any situation, no matter how hard, we have decisions to make, either wrong, right or undecided. Indecision is a decision. This power is needed concerning our health, especially on how we respond to stress. Although stress can be positive in some cases, especially when it helps us avoid danger or meet deadlines. Stress can be described as a feeling of emotional or physical tension. It is our response to threats in any given situation. On the other hand, when there is a sustained mental health disorder that is triggered by stress is known as anxiety. Stress can erupt from any form or thoughts that make us feel nervous, frustrated, or angry. This is the way our body reacts to demands or challenges.

Perpetually condoning stress is never a good way to have a healthy life because it will eventually puncture the balloon of one's good immune system, which will make someone vulnerable to Illnesses. Cultivating the habit that walks away from frustration, trouble, anger, and anxiety is one of the ways to keep our body healthy. Some other ways are:

1. Accept that there are situations that you cannot control.

2. Keeping a positive attitude always.

3. Exercise regularly.

4. Replace aggression with an assertion.

5. Learn relaxation techniques like meditation, etc.

6. Eat a healthy and well-balanced meal.

The above list is a way to keep the physical body in shape. However, the word of God through the Apostle Paul to us in the book of **Philippians 4:6-9** states that:

"Be anxious for nothing, but in everything by prayer and supplication, with thanksgivings, let your requests be made known to God; and the peace of God, which surpasses all understanding, will guard your hearts and mind through Christ Jesus".

This means that even God is aware that we will have reasons to have anxiety but has warned us to be anxious for nothing whatsoever. Instead, we are encouraged to tender anything that bothers us before God to help us fix it with an assurance that the peace of God will guard our mind when we do it.

Many people major on minor and get frustrated along the line, but it is wiser to consider God first. What is it that can bother us so much that will shift our mind from the Almighty, simply to frighten and prepare us for its torment? The way to truly have freedom from stress, worry, fear, anger, anxiety, etc. is to focus on God. The book of Galatians 5:19-23 gives some fantastic exposition on two categories we all belong and what it may trigger. It states:

1. The acts of flesh are obvious: sexual immorality, impurity and debauchery;

2. Idolatry and witchcraft; hatred, discord, jealousy, fits of rage, selfish ambition, dissensions, factions.

3. And envy; drunkenness, orgies, and the like. I warn you, as i did before, that those who live like this will not inherit the kingdom of God.

4. But the fruit of the Spirit is love, joy, peace, forbearance, kindness, goodness, faithfulness,

5. Gentleness and self-control. Against such things there is no law.

Starting from verse 19, it says the acts of the flesh "are" obvious, which means, they are many and can be carried out by different people. It is surprising to know that all acts of the flesh will, in one way or the other, cause illness to our physical health.

There is no one that has jealousy, hatred, fits of rage, selfish ambition, faction, dissension, envy that can ever know peace. This is because the people having such acts will have a lot to bother about, keep malice, and have many people to fight. The people who have this act are not far from stress and anxiety, which is detrimental to their health, not forgetting that the Bible warns against it also. Another thing to understand is that anyone that operates in any of these acts has the works of the flesh in action in his life.

The works of the spirit can only manifest in a person that has given himself to God, and God has, in turn, taken over of such person, then the fruits of the Spirit that we may see as the attributes of God now manifest in human. While the fruits of the Spirit are great and can keep you in good health in your physical body, it helps spiritually to live in God's manifestations and be carriers of His fruits. To live in the Spirit, you have to be intentional about it so that all the friends that will not be needed on that path can get a notification from now.

Power of Choice:

One of the greatest gifts from God to humanity is giving us the power to make choices. Each time we make a choice, we exercise our power to decide what to do, when, where, and how to do it. The amazing part of it is the aspect of indecision and its effect.

Do not be surprised if I tell you that you may make the right decision or a wrong one, but your hesitation that falls in-between is equally your decision. The outcome of your indecision is as bad as your wrong decision because the expectation is towards your right decision.

Your decision to shun the lifestyle that endangers your life today will turn a lot of things about you around. Considering how detrimental some lifestyles are to your health today is a day to quit alcohol and your smoking habit. Not only that, anything you do that opens up your immune system to vulnerability should be stopped, now that your system is still doing well. It is also a very good time to enjoy God's growth by feeding at his table daily, where you will be able to decree what you want into reality. When we allow God's influence over our life, we allow ourselves to be plugged to the source of all existing things and enjoy his promises to those who care to follow him. By consuming God's words daily, we will become more of Him when we follow all that is written, especially when the fruits of the Spirit begin to manifest.

Dear friend, your decision to fortify your immune system is better started in the spiritual because we control the physical from the spiritual. Building a serious relationship with God is the right decision that will not only help you beyond the medical and physical here on earth but till eternity. Even when our bodies get more attacks from illnesses as we are aging, our spirits will remain intact with the source of all strengths that shed abroad His unconditional love to anyone who decides to follow Him. And while the spirit of such an aged person departs, it will be eternity face to face with the creator in His paradise. Tell me, would you be invited to live eternally in a paradise that belongs to someone you have not built a stable relationship with? No! Another beautiful thing about choice making is that you are always sure what end will be on the path you have chosen, and that is why you are getting this today.

There are victories that you can only get when you go spiritual, especially those that torment people physically from the spiritual realm. Your immunity (spiritual immunity) in this situation can only be God in every sense of it. This is when you can say what is written in the book of Galatians 6:17 that "from henceforth let no man trouble me: for I bear in my body the marks of the Lord Jesus." That is the immunity because the trouble may be sickness, viruses, insanity, or any demonic affliction. All of these can only be achieved through God's unconditional love.

Unconditional Love:

The book of John 3:16 mention the sincere love of God for all mankind, such that before you desire to think of loving God, He has loved you. A songwriter describes God's love by saying:

"Could we with ink the ocean fill and were the skies of parchment made;

Were every stalk of earth a quill and every man a scribe by trade;

To write the love of God above would drain the ocean dry..."

It is referred to as an unconditional love because of its overflowing and relentless efforts towards a season of picking unfaithful men. Unconditional love is devoid of fear and fallacy in all situations that, despite being ignored by men, He still doesn't want the death of any winner. Although God is love personified, the love of God is Jesus, given as a gift unto all men, crucified, bled to death, buried, and resurrected on the third day. That was when love went on the cross and bled mercy for everyone who will accept Him. When you accept God's love, your eternity with God in heaven is certain. That is why that passage says, "Whosoever believes in Him shall not perish but have eternal life." When you called Jesus into your life there is a strong need to live in the consciousness of who you are now.

Forgiveness

Forgiveness seems to be the toughest thing to do, depending on the committed offenses. Something happened between Jesus and one of his disciples Peter in Mathew 18:21-22: Then Peter came to Jesus and asked, "Lord, how many times shall I forgive my brother or sister who sins against me? Up to seven times?" 22 Jesus answered, "I tell you, not seven times, but seventy-seven times. This is simply teaching us to let go in several cases of offense towards us, and by these, we will free ourselves from anger and troubles.

When you are offended, and you fail to forgive, you are the one that will suffer the most because the offense hurts, and keeping it (unforgiving) is worse. Another thing to see is that, when people hurt you, whether they apologize or not, they keep on living their lives but you keep living in the yesterday of what was done to you such that each time you meet or they look back, they still see you there. Please, my friend, move on.

Letting go is what God does each time we apologize for whatever we do wrong. Let us consider how Psalms 103:12 put it: "As far as the east is from the west, so far hath he removed our transgressions from us." God keeps moving on so you too should. And when you ask God for the forgiveness of any sin, and you repent, believe that you are forgiven because God works with your sincerity and the intent of your heart.

Faith

The only lifeline that makes a man walk with God is faith. "Faith is the substance of things hoped for, evidence of things not seen" according to Hebrew 11:1, and this means our lives should not be based on only visible things. When we trust God that we cannot see, it is faith. When we accept Jesus that died and resurrected over 2000 years ago as our Lord and savior, inviting him into our lives may sincerely look stupid to normal human reasoning, but that is faith.

Believing that what you do not have now, you will not lack in the future by God's provision is faith. When you pray to God that you do not see, but you believe is in heaven, is faith. With faith, impossibility is possible and exploits that come to be in a way far beyond your reasoning. I encourage you today to have faith in God as you follow Him and watch Him heal, deliver, set free and meet your needs. When you pray, you should constantly tell God about your health from what you desire and what shouldn't occur. So, pray in the name of Jesus to God in heaven and believe without doubts or fear, even when it is the toughest moment that everything around you is indicating that your prayers will not be answered. Don't forget that God responds faster to a prayer of faith as well as a man of faith.

NEW BIRTH CONSCIOUSNESS

Now that you have been called out of darkness into God's marvelous light as a new creature, it is highly important to begin to live in the reality of who you are. Just like when a slave has been set free, he becomes as free as his master, enjoys every liberty of his former boss. In reality, however, the lifestyle of a slave roams in his consciousness such that, when he has all the right to act, he is still afraid in his mind. Jesus says in John 8:36 that "If the Son, therefore, shall make you free, ye shall be free indeed."

There is freedom for everyone that comes under the umbrella of Jesus, and every one of such people must learn how to live in that reality. This same thing is what the Apostle Paul through the Holy Ghost was telling the Corinthians in 2 Corinthians 5:17 that "therefore if any man be in Christ, he is a new creature: old things have passed away; behold all things has become new." At this point, there is no more living in your yesterday; instead, hold on and view the better days ahead, while you live in the now. This time, your bad life has gone with your old, sinful, wicked life. You are now God's direct son with whom He can keep communicating with as long as He likes when you are available to hear Him.

Eternal Life

Our days on this planet are numbered, and we will pass on to the life beyond. There are two eternal lives:

1. Eternal life with God

2. Eternal life in Hell

We all have the choice to choose now, where we want our eternal life to be.

1. Eternal life with God: This is where everyone that accept Jesus Christ as their Lord and savior and follows Him truthfully will end up. They will see Jesus in His glory because they would have been translated from this mortal body into an immortal celestial one. Only those whose names are found written in the book of life will find their place with God. Those who have the acts of flesh will not have their place in heaven. Revelation 3:5 states: "The one who is victorious will, like them, be dressed in white. I will never blot out the name of that person from the book of life, but will acknowledge that name before my Father and his angels."

Heaven is where all saints will be rewarded to have eternal bliss for trusting in God through thick and thin.

2. Eternal life in Hell: This is where those whose names are not found in the book of life will be punished eternally.

1 Corinthians 6:9-10 says

"9. Or do you not know that wrongdoers will not inherit the kingdom of God? Do not be deceived: Neither the sexually immoral nor idolaters nor adulterers nor men who have sex with men 10. nor thieves nor the greedy nor drunkards nor slanderers nor swindlers will inherit the kingdom of God."

In another passage, it states clearly that those who are liars and doers of other acts listed in the acts of flesh mentioned above will not have a place in heaven. Revelation 20:15 "anyone whose name was not found written in the book of life was thrown into the lake of fire."

21-DAY IMMUNE SYSTEM TRACKER CHALLENGE

The **GOAL** is to **APPLY** a maximum of these immune system boosters in your body every single day. Ready to go…. **Go!**

1. Citrus fruits

2. Red Bell peppers

3. Broccoli

4. Garlic

5. Ginger

6. Spinach

7. Yogurt

8. Almonds

9. Sunflower seeds

10. Turmeric

11. Green Tea

12. Papaya

13. Kiwi

14. Poultry

15. Shellfish

16. Blueberries

17. Dark chocolate

18. Sweet Potatoes

19. Salmon

20. Sleep

21. Exercise

22. Socializing

23. Attitude

24. Soul Food (inspiring words)

25. Groove Smile (everyday)

21- Day Immune System Tracker Challenge

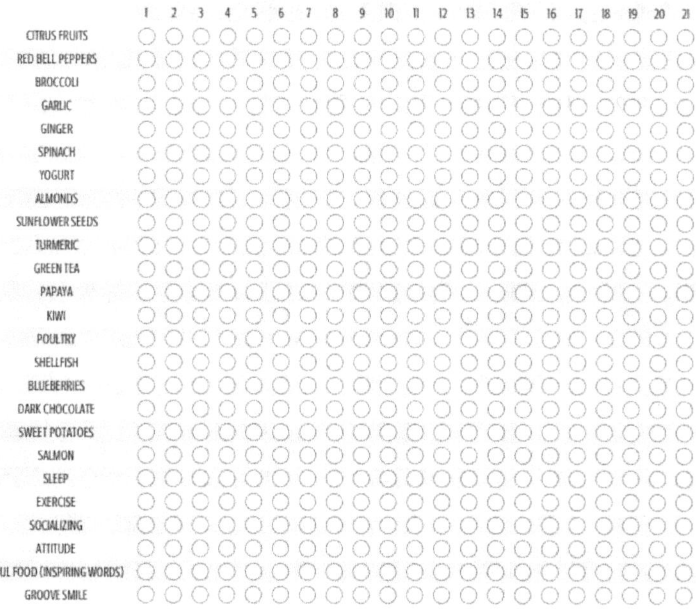

THE **GOAL** IS TO **APPLY** A MAXIMUM OF THESE IMMUNE SYSTEM BOOSTERS IN YOUR BODY EVERY SINGLE DAY. READY TO GO.... **GO!**

	1	2	3	4	5	6	7	8	9	10	11	12	13	14	15	16	17	18	19	20	21
CITRUS FRUITS	○	○	○	○	○	○	○	○	○	○	○	○	○	○	○	○	○	○	○	○	○
RED BELL PEPPERS	○	○	○	○	○	○	○	○	○	○	○	○	○	○	○	○	○	○	○	○	○
BROCCOLI	○	○	○	○	○	○	○	○	○	○	○	○	○	○	○	○	○	○	○	○	○
GARLIC	○	○	○	○	○	○	○	○	○	○	○	○	○	○	○	○	○	○	○	○	○
GINGER	○	○	○	○	○	○	○	○	○	○	○	○	○	○	○	○	○	○	○	○	○
SPINACH	○	○	○	○	○	○	○	○	○	○	○	○	○	○	○	○	○	○	○	○	○
YOGURT	○	○	○	○	○	○	○	○	○	○	○	○	○	○	○	○	○	○	○	○	○
ALMONDS	○	○	○	○	○	○	○	○	○	○	○	○	○	○	○	○	○	○	○	○	○
SUNFLOWER SEEDS	○	○	○	○	○	○	○	○	○	○	○	○	○	○	○	○	○	○	○	○	○
TURMERIC	○	○	○	○	○	○	○	○	○	○	○	○	○	○	○	○	○	○	○	○	○
GREEN TEA	○	○	○	○	○	○	○	○	○	○	○	○	○	○	○	○	○	○	○	○	○
PAPAYA	○	○	○	○	○	○	○	○	○	○	○	○	○	○	○	○	○	○	○	○	○
KIWI	○	○	○	○	○	○	○	○	○	○	○	○	○	○	○	○	○	○	○	○	○
POULTRY	○	○	○	○	○	○	○	○	○	○	○	○	○	○	○	○	○	○	○	○	○
SHELLFISH	○	○	○	○	○	○	○	○	○	○	○	○	○	○	○	○	○	○	○	○	○
BLUEBERRIES	○	○	○	○	○	○	○	○	○	○	○	○	○	○	○	○	○	○	○	○	○
DARK CHOCOLATE	○	○	○	○	○	○	○	○	○	○	○	○	○	○	○	○	○	○	○	○	○
SWEET POTATOES	○	○	○	○	○	○	○	○	○	○	○	○	○	○	○	○	○	○	○	○	○
SALMON	○	○	○	○	○	○	○	○	○	○	○	○	○	○	○	○	○	○	○	○	○
SLEEP	○	○	○	○	○	○	○	○	○	○	○	○	○	○	○	○	○	○	○	○	○
EXERCISE	○	○	○	○	○	○	○	○	○	○	○	○	○	○	○	○	○	○	○	○	○
SOCIALIZING	○	○	○	○	○	○	○	○	○	○	○	○	○	○	○	○	○	○	○	○	○
ATTITUDE	○	○	○	○	○	○	○	○	○	○	○	○	○	○	○	○	○	○	○	○	○
SOUL FOOD (INSPIRING WORDS)	○	○	○	○	○	○	○	○	○	○	○	○	○	○	○	○	○	○	○	○	○
GROOVE SMILE	○	○	○	○	○	○	○	○	○	○	○	○	○	○	○	○	○	○	○	○	○

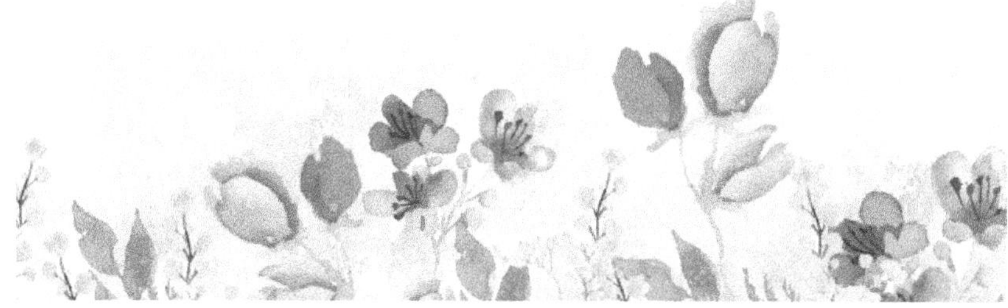

CONCLUSION

To conclude, I encourage you today to make a decision to invest in your physical and spiritual immune system. Choose to balance your 7 dimensions of life. If you need some introduction to the 7 dimensions of life, make sure you get your copy of

"The Rainbow Lifestyle Blueprint ". If you balance your 7 dimensions of life, you'll attain a peaceful lifestyle from the inside.

Other great inspiring program resources on Amazon by GLADYS GLOBAL:

- Mind And Body Fitness program

- Spiritual And Soul Fitness

- True Wealth And Financial Fitness

- Corona Word

- Passion Tracker

- The Rainbow Lifestyle Blueprint